What Every Young Man Should Know About Sex

But few ever learn

By Marvin Lee Robey

What Every Young Man Should Know
About Sex

And Few Ever Learn

Copy Right: Marvin Lee Robey

What Every Young Man Should Know
About Sex

Second Edition

Print ISBN 978-0-9798556-6-5

Electronic ISBN 978-0-9798556-5-8

Library of Congress Control Number
2012906476

Published June 2012

DEDICATION

This book is dedicated to the Second Sexual Revolution

Most of us have seen the First Sexual Revolution in which we gained the now common sexual freedom.

This book is dedicated to the Second Sexual Revolution with the simple, common practice of women enjoying sex as much as any man while the man's pleasure is increased with the illusive mutual orgasm with her, even if she has never been able to have an orgasm before.

INTRODUCTION

This book gives a young man the knowledge to move gradually from a passionate kiss into full sex including the illusive mutual orgasm with the caressing and the sex blended together so smoothly there is no real distinction.

Although he is leading her all the way, she is actually leading him in her feminine way.

By the end of the mutual orgasm she will have experienced two strong orgasms in two distinct parts of her body.

Also Introducing Extended Love,

giving the man increased pleasure while easily giving the woman continuous orgasms as long as she wants.

CONTENTS

CONTENTS

Chapter 1

SEX AND LOVE

Contrary to general understanding, humans are unlike any other creature in the matter of sex. Unlike all other animals, humans practice sex regardless of the female being "in heat". Furthermore, unlike animals and men, women have more than one area of their body through which they experience the heights of sexual pleasure. In fact a healthy woman's whole body becomes a sex organ when she is raised to passion.

She seldom enjoys sex when done the way most men do it, only thinking of how animals do it and THEY THINK they themselves like it. They then assume if she does not like it something is wrong with her. These common assumptions are based upon what seems logical to him, but is not based upon an informed point of view of what she needs or they themselves actually want.

Most men want to do it in fifteen minutes and it is done. Only about one third of all women have any orgasm that way, which is her real pleasure. Even if she does, it is almost always cut so short as to leave her disappointed. If it is so important to men, why are they in such a hurry to finish it? Why not take the time to really enjoy the experience of it?

This book will show you how to give the average woman a series of strong orgasms with a high level of pleasure flowing through three different areas of her body, each feeling very different from the last and continually changing until she is exhausted if she wants and you will take the time and effort. It will also show you how you can increase your pleasure, although no man can come close to the pleasure she is capable of experiencing.

This book will also teach you to give her two strong and complete, but different orgasms in 35 minutes and show you how to achieve the illusive mutual orgasm which will further increase both of your pleasures every time.

The vast pleasure a woman can naturally experience from sex makes it a huge lose to most women for men to be so lacking in the knowledge of how to best please both the woman and even himself.

This lack of knowledge also leads to much discord between men and women. Or, the actual knowledge can lead to a woman who is absolutely yours.

Very few women are aware of these capabilities of theirs, but if a man is leading, she does not need to know. She just wants to relax and enjoy it all.

History records a very few men who commanded an extreme attraction of women, such as Casanova. Although much of their appeal was always their personality, this book gives you their secrets in bed.

There must be a reason for these differences between humans and animals.

Those who have seen animals do it and therefore think they know how to please a woman or experience the most from it themselves are badly mistaken.

We can easily discern the obvious reason for having two sexes, and the constant attraction between them in humans by studying the only sexual practices that really give pleasure to both men and especially women.

When we experience the love of a mate, the whole world seems brighter and others around us seem more likeable.

By sharing physical pleasures, we learn to love each other and this love expands our love for all of mankind.

Generally speaking, men want sex. Women want love. They are coming from opposite directions and until the two meet in the middle, there will be conflict. Yet both want the same thing that is only found in the middle and neither will be fully satisfied until the two do meet there. Love is the other half of the equation for men. Sex is the other half of the equation for women. But neither one can just have their half. They are actually seeking the others half. The purpose of physical intimacy is for each to experience the other missing part of themselves. They must be combined.

Sex is given to us to draw us together in love and teach us to love. It is teaching us of the other half that is missing from us. If we think we are complete in ourselves and do not need the other half we are deluding ourselves. The more we learn to appreciate and understand the opposite sex the more we will feel complete in ourselves.

We must learn to enjoy giving others pleasure, instead of the constant conflict we are commonly engaged in through jealousy, greed, hatred, ignorance, suspicion and laziness to get only what we want, or think we want. We need to learn to work with one another in a win-win practice and enjoy harmony and helping others.

Once a man has learned to take the time and effort to give a woman the pleasure she is capable of experiencing, and really needs, and he experiences the pleasure of doing so, he is a long step further in understanding love of life itself. Only love brings us lasting pleasure. Sex without love is shallow and leaves both partners feeling something is missing, as it is. What is missing is love. Love of one thing leads us to love all things.

But "love" is not just sex. Sex is only the outward, physical expression of love. Love is an emotion. Sex is physical. Only when the physical act is done as an expression of the emotion of love does sex become "making love".

Even with the subject of sex taught in the schools, it is amazing how many young girls have no knowledge of the dangers of pregnancy related to it. Most young girls today have heard of the "pill", but still have little knowledge of the subject and many are easily seduced with no protection without comprehending what is happening.

They enjoy a good kiss. Going further with it is very pleasant and no harm comes from it. But she does not know there is a place where a danger line exists or just why. Something is feeling good, so it must be good. She often does not know what is happening. Sex is continually portrayed in the movies and television as irresistible and common and safe. The only consideration is; is the partner "sexy"?

The old theory seems to be: "If they don't know anything about it, they will not be curious about it and will not know the subject even exists and therefore they will not have a problem." History clearly shows this theory has never worked. If parents will think back to when they were teenagers they will know that. With the broad exposure to sex today, that concept has become ridiculous. Only knowledge can protect them.

Women have always wanted a man who has a broad knowledge of women, including sex. Throughout history men have usually wanted women who have never had sex before and know little about men or sex. If a woman has had sex before, they might have had a better experience than with their present lover and that would be a problem. If they have not had sex before they will not know the difference.

These two concepts are not compatible. Who are men to gain this knowledge from? Their parents withhold what little they know of the subject. Churches have generally related it with sin. They are not likely to gain it from prostitutes. They naturally think once they have copied animals and performed it a couple of times they now know just about all that is important. If they want to know more they buy a book on a doctor's description of anatomy and the dangers of disease or a book on the hundred or so acrobatic sex positions, kinky sex, or

Chinese routines which very few would ever want to try and none of which increase either partners' actual pleasure.

Even after reading a dozen of these books they still do not know the basics of sex. They feel something is missing, but they are looking in the wrong places. Until they realize there are basics they do not understand, they will never learn and there will be discord between men and women in both love and sex and this will probably lead to other discord between them.

We see many men described as very sexy who are really a bit ugly. Why are they considered sexy? Largely because they portray confidence in life and with women. They are worldly. Therefore it appears, they probably know women and understand love and sex. This confidence usually comes from enough knowledge, and ease relating to women to attract women's desire to experience more of them. If you want to be "sexy", you will have to become knowledgeable about women and at ease with them. To be at ease with women you must understand them. Women naturally gravitate to men who are at ease with women. Other men struggle to win a woman.

Knowing about sex is like knowing anything else. There are four stages to knowing anything:

The first stage is; you don't know you don't know. This stage is hard to pass because you don't even know there is something you need to know. It is almost impossible to learn anything from this position. This is where most men are. Making matters even worse, they have decided they know everything of importance of love and sex, and have thereby blocked out any further knowledge of the subject.

The second stage is; you know you don't know. Now you have a good chance of learning.

The third stage is; you know.

The fourth stage is; you know you know. This can only come as a certainty from within.

Unfortunately, most men are in the first stage and many women are too, even of their own selves. Most men have blocked out any further knowledge of the subject, both from a belief they know all there is to know and/or from their ego telling them that to be a man they must know all about sex, therefore they must defend their position of knowing.

So, open your mind a short while, at least to yourself, where you do not have to defend your competence to anyone and examine the concepts in this book. Then you will be able to face the world with genuine confidence.

In as much as it is natural for men to give women sexual pleasure while the woman just relaxes and enjoys it, women do not really need to know much about it, if the man does. All she has to do is accept the pleasures he is giving her. If he is continually giving her pleasure, she only wants more. She is not interested in serving your needs.

She certainly is not interested in a hundred strenuous positions such as standing on her head! She wants to completely relax and experience the pleasures. Actually, she usually does not really know what she likes until she experiences it.

The man has to know what she needs and wants, even when she does not know. Then he has to know how to give it to her. He often does not even know what he really wants or how to get it, much less what she wants. And she often does not know what she wants either, until she gets it. Even then she may not know nor care what happened.

It is very common for a man to roll off of a woman, dress in a hurry, head down to his hang out at the local bar, swagger in and laughingly say to his buddies: "Man, did I fuck her good!" So what is he laughing about? And when her girl friend comes over and asks what is wrong she says: "Oh, John fucked me again." "Didn't you like it?" "Hell, no!" "Well, why do you do it then?" "Oh, that's what he expects." What a poor excuse!

John thinks he is a real man, or he is trying to believe it, and this proves it and he is manly in being able to coerce her into it and really give it to her. He will not subconsciously feel good about himself or the experience. She has not responded with even a smile, much less a warm hug, a passionate kiss or warm word.

If she did not like it, that must be her fault. It certainly is not his. He did a good job. How could he have done any better? He does not know. So he must find new victims to conquer, looking for a woman who enjoys it and makes him feel like he really did a good job. His best bet is in finding a woman who will fake it.

Men talk and joke to their buddies and even to women constantly about sex and see how it is done in the movies including the explicit porno movies and if there were anything of importance they didn't know they would have found out by now; or so they think.

But the jokes are mostly based upon ignorance and suppositions. So are the movies. In the porno movies, the woman appears to always be quickly reaching an orgasm, usually instantly. In real life she seldom ever reaches an orgasm or if she does it is ended almost as soon as it starts. She's just faking it.

What really makes this a very sad situation is that most men never do learn any more than the rudiments all of their life. Furthermore, the women are strongly influenced subconsciously by their first experience that is usually unpleasant, because the guy just did not know how to make it a pleasant experience. Thus many women who could find much more pleasure in sex to enjoy, even much more than men, quickly decide they do not like it and that they are just being used by men, which is probably true.

Once a woman's subconscious mind accepts the concept that sex is unpleasant and men are just using them, they may never learn to enjoy it, even from a really good lover. The subconscious mind turns what it labels pleasant into joy, but what it labels as unpleasant it turns into just that. If it labels it as pressure, then it is pressure, if it labels it as hot, it is hot, if it labels it as cold, it is cold, if it labels it as pain, then it is pain.

For instance, many women describe the pains of childbirth as the most painful experience possible, while other women find childbirth little problem under hypnosis and without the tension of fear, deliver much quicker and more safely, without anesthesia of herself and the baby. The difference is what the subconscious mind has labeled it. This has been proven over and over again. It is what the subconscious labels it.

When a growing girl has heard her mother and her mothers' friends talking about the horrible pains of childbirth and then as a woman her gynecologist reinforces that concept, childbirth will be much more painful than if she had never heard the subject discussed. This is generally known as the placebo effect. Once the subconscious mind labels something, it is difficult to change it, and it will be experienced as the subconscious has labeled it.

If a man comes along later who could give a woman real pleasure, and her first experience was unpleasant, she may have already turned her subconscious mind against it. That is one reason why it is so important that a girls' first experience should be good.

Almost all men like sex. Only about three-fourths of women are capable of enjoying it. Even those will seldom enjoy their first few experiences. If we realize that women have the capacity to enjoy sex far more than any man can, this is a very sad fact. There are probably ninety-nine women out of a hundred who never find out what a huge and wonderful capacity for pleasure they have, in all of their life. It is a rare man indeed who will even believe women have this capacity.

The best time to learn how to give this to a woman is before your first experience of sex. If you have already had sex, whether you are a teenager or sixty years old, the best time to learn is now. It is essential that you get the real knowledge of sex and love when you are young, before you have given up. If you do you will have few problems in life with women.

I think that by the time you have finished reading this book you will understand how most women can enjoy sex much more than any man and that it is a pleasure for her lover to give it to her. She cannot do it herself. Both the man and the woman will then feel good about themselves and their relationship.

In this book you will find out how to have her always wanting more and leading you to it instead of resisting it. But although she must lead you, you must first lead her. This may seem like a contradiction, but I will make this clear as you read on. I have no doubt that many young men would want to have such a relationship with the woman they love.

When a man first meets a new lover, he has a strong desire to see and touch her nude body all over. Most women love to have the right man touch them all over as much as he wants to or more.

Many men have sex with a woman and yet never touch most parts of her body. And yet, isn't it more enjoyable to both look at it and touch it than to just look at it? It is so soft, shapely, smooth and alive. And she loves to be touched all over. She enjoys the intimacy. And she likes to feel your body too. No, strange as it may seem, sex is not the primary experience of intimacy.

Without this loving of her body, she will not be ready for intercourse. You will have to use your own lubricant and she will dislike the sex.

By the time you have finished this book these differences will no longer be a problem or a mystery. By the time you have finished this book, you will understand the ancient mystery of the differences between men and women. You will also be able to establish a truly close relationship with the woman of your choice. You will both enjoy each other and be able to communicate easily with one another in order to continue to increase that mutual pleasure and all aspects of your relationship. You will both feel good about it afterward instead of the common feeling that something is not right or something is missing.

CHAPTER 2

ANATOMY

The first thing you need to know is where are the parts of a woman related to her pleasures that are not obvious. That is the subject of this short chapter. Looking at the figure on the next page illustrating a cross section of a woman's genital organs as described in the following chapters, you can find:

1. The pubic bone which protects the genital organs much like in men.
2. Vagina
3. Clitoris
4. Uterus
5. Cervix
6. G-spot
7. Labia Minora
8. Labia Majora

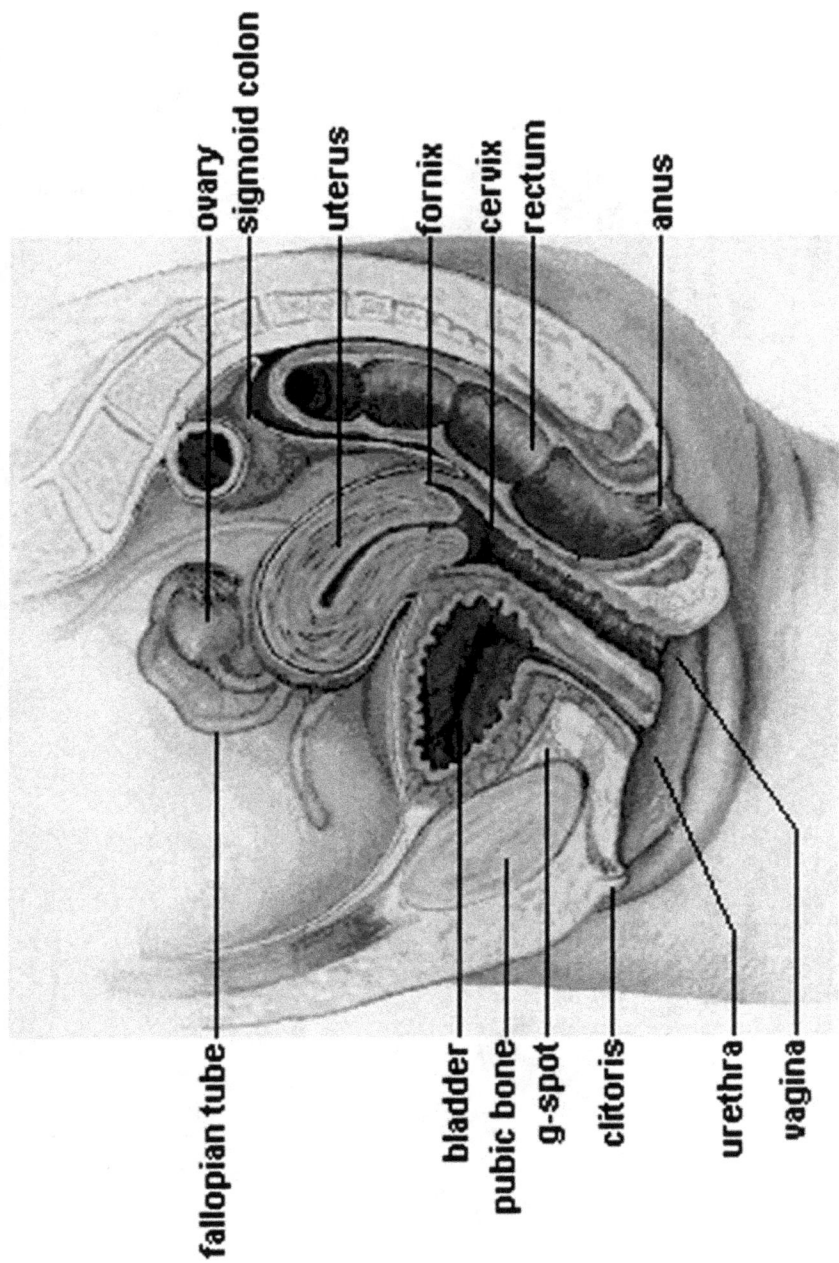

ovary
sigmoid colon
uterus
fornix
cervix
rectum
anus

fallopian tube
bladder
pubic bone
g-spot
clitoris
urethra
vagina

CHAPTER 3

THE DIFFERENCES BETWEEN MEN AND WOMEN

From the beginning of history, men have considered women to be an unsolvable mystery. And women have likewise complained about not understanding men. This has been the source of much conflict, as well as much attraction between them. You probably have noticed some differences and like what you see in women, or you would not be reading this book. Men and women are obviously physically different. Their personalities are also different.

To think their bodies are all the differences there are between them is a bad mistake. Boys and girls are raised together, educated together and required to pass the same academic tests. But women will usually excel in different subjects than men will. Furthermore, men and women will often learn some subjects in a different manner if allowed to. They tend to approach understanding and knowledge from different directions. For instance, in mathematics, women will usually learn by memorizing the subject, while men try to reason out the subject. In languages, women memorize the words, and judge what looks right, while men look for a formula for the language. This is not always true, as there are many differences between different men and there are many differences between different women, but it is generally true.

Women who tend to approach subjects from a more logical point of view will often approach sex from more nearly a man's point of view. These differences may be helpful to you in understanding the differences among the women you know.

Consider a man and a woman in a grocery store or clothing store for example. A man wants to know where everything is and wants to go right to it and buy it. He is irritated when it has been moved or the label changed. He wants it to look exactly the same as it did the last time he bought it and be where it was. A woman wants to shop and look at everything. If everything has been moved, she enjoys the challenge of finding it. It is now a riddle; a game. She wants things that are different from what she has seen before. She spots things she is looking for quicker than a man.

One of the common pleasures of a woman is to go shopping. Even if she has no money, she loves to spend an afternoon "window shopping". It is a well known fact that women's items cost more than men's because the salesmen must spend considerably more time with women to make a sale than they would with men and that time costs the store more money. Furthermore, women often buy on a whim but later change their mind and return what they bought. This is expensive to a store. Women enjoy all of this. Thus women's clothing is more expensive than men's.

Many women have no concept of money or debt and you may not be able to explain it to her. If a woman is given a way to purchase things she wants she will do so. Thus credit cards and lay aways. When she is confronted with unpaid, overdue bills she will often seriously reply; "But its only money." If she is working and paying the bills herself, this will still be her serious reply.

Does this mean she is just plain dumb? No! She may be very intelligent and understand many things that few men understand. There are other ways of knowing other than logic and being told or taught things.

All of this does not apply to all women, of course. From one woman to another, there is as much difference as night and day, just as there is in men. Isn't that one of the things that make women so interesting? But by understanding this as a common difference in women and men and realizing it is basically female and the difference is basically degrees of these qualities, you will understand women much better.

If a man only goes through a rudimentary, mechanical sex act, he will enjoy it. She seldom will. She will just be getting started when he is finished.

Both before and especially after sex, she wants to be held close and talk and be loved. He is leaving. Her attitude is: "No more of that!" Now he wonders why. If she didn't enjoy it, it's her fault. Actually, if he understood women, he would know it is actually his fault.

Until he learns to enjoy a woman's body properly, so that she is CONCIOUSLY GIVING him the experience and sharing in his pleasure AND HE IN HERS, he is missing most of the potential pleasure, and she is very likely missing all of it. Most of his pleasure can only come from his loving her whole being and expressing it clearly; her personality, her soft skin, so alive, the many wonderful, beautiful curves of her body, and the pleasure of seeing and feeling them lasts so much longer than the sex act. And it's always good to experience again and share her pleasure of it.

She will only enjoy the sex experience when she can fully enjoy her whole body and her whole self being loved, not just one little part of it and she loves to touch your body too; your tough hard body with its hard muscles, as well as your personality. Talking is a sharing of your personalities, which should be the strongest attraction between you. This is not separate from the love between you which leads to the sex act.

Nothing pleases a woman so much as that which makes her feel good about herself. Isn't this true of men too? If your lovemaking makes her feel inadequate, inferior or used for any reason, you loose. If you make her feel good about herself in every way; her personality as well as her body, you will almost always win. Try to find what she feels is her weakness and try to strengthen it and you will almost always win.

Women need to be loved and their bodies do too. Those are two different things. That may seem difficult to understand. Many areas of psychiatry have shown beyond a doubt that women who have an unsatisfactory sex life have health problems related to it and some become serious. To some extent, physical sex and the loving of her body are two very different things. In another way, they are the same thing.

Loving a women's body is not just admiring it from a distance. Her whole body needs to be touched in a loving manner and different parts need to be touched differently, but always lovingly, as though it were the most precious thing in the world; and it almost is, isn't it? This is not just an emotional need, it is also a physical need and is necessary to her physical health.

She first wants her personality to be loved. Then she wants her body to be physically loved. From there sex naturally develops. She wants sex, but it must come in this order.

A man must first learn that, no matter how much a woman enjoys sex, when she is not actively involved in it, her mind is seldom on the subject. For instance, if she takes a roller coaster ride, she may intensely enjoy it, but an hour later it is momentarily forgotten. To her, sex is the same way. A man cannot forget about sex however, because his body continually reminds him of it. Hers does not. He must remind her of it in little ways and as often as possible to prepare her for coming sex.

However, until they have experienced sex together, some women will be offended and really turned off by any flirtation except a carefully directed flirtation expressing love. Her desire for sex only comes after loving her whole body. That comes in stages and sequences

AFTER SHE IS READY FOR EACH SEPARATE PART OF HER BODY TO BE LOVED, BUT NOT UNTIL THEN.

Acceptance of touching her body must come in the proper sequence. Just as with all of us, what we consider our space can only be invaded under the right conditions. What we consider our space changes as our situation changes. We want friends in what would be an invasion of our space by strangers. In love making, what she considers her space changes as she accepts other moves into her space. Once she has accepted you into all the areas of her body, she is now yours. But not until then. To really make her yours, you must love her whole body, a part at a time.

I will discuss how to remind her of sex in chapter 6.

A man generally thinks of sex primarily through the sex organs. Few women do. Sex brings women and men together in love. That is Natures way.

There would be no reason to have two sexes if it were not for men and women to learn of the relationship of the physical to the emotional. Man teaches woman to understand the physical. Woman teaches man to understand the emotional. To most men, "love" is primarily a very materialistic thing and generally centers around the sex organs. To most women, it is not materialistic at all. To women it must come as an expression of love from the heart. It centers around love.

She will tell you flowers are romantic. Love poems are romantic. A beautiful secluded hideaway perfect for lovers is romantic. It is a beautiful place for love. An only slightly different secluded love nest may be embarrassing and offensive if it is directly related to sex. If its purpose appears to be for sex, it is offensive. If its purpose appears to be for love it is romantic. If love is the central issue with the emotions coming first, it is beautiful.

To a woman, love is first of all an emotion. It can be very well expressed as sex, with strong physical sensations being given through love. To a woman, her whole being must be involved including her whole body AND her emotions. It is necessary for her to feel the man's pleasures are coming through her. It is her love he is feeling, and enjoying and she is giving it to him. She needs to feel it is his love she is feeling as sexual pleasure. The sexual pleasures she is feeling flow from a concentration of the love he is giving her.

She should not notice any sudden change from making love to her body to actual sex. It should be a smooth transition, or perhaps not a transition but only a continuous increase of pleasure throughout. She must have this close feeling between them. These must be her messages to and from her subconscious mind.

To a man, sex is usually very physical. He is quite ready to do it and get it over with. However, if he will take the time and trouble to do it her way, he will soon find he has been missing much of the pleasure he could have had, and the very personal, and beautiful relationship that comes with it. It is probably largely her personality that has really attracted him to her. If he takes sex in the manner most men do, he is missing the interaction with her personality, which is much of the pleasure he could be receiving. He is missing her responses to him. These responses are the pleasures coming from her personality during love making. They should be much of his pleasure.

A man is usually first attracted to a woman by certain qualities of her body he finds very desirable. Her breasts; her small waist, her hair and other qualities. Maybe her neck or her back, her legs, her lips. He may soon find certain qualities of her personality even more desirable. But most men do not experience these qualities in her when thinking of sex. He wants to go straight to sex. He sees no reason why he should physically express his admiration of these qualities. Why should he when she already knows how attractive she is to him? To a woman, the love of her whole being needs to be loved both verbally, visually and physically. Does he really find her whole being, including her personality attractive or only her sex organs? She knows her sex organs are probably not that different from most other women's, and if they are he does not know that to begin with. If it is her personality and her body in general that has attracted him, why is he only interested in her sex organs?

If he takes his pleasure without expressing his love for her whole being in every way, she feels cheated, fucked or almost as though she had been raped. "All he wants is sex." She needs to know she is not just any woman to him but someone very special. If a man will take the time to admire and enjoy the details he loves her for each time he makes love to her, and hopefully at times in between, both will have a much closer and pleasant relationship. He will probably find he enjoys all of it and the whole experience much more.

CHAPTER 4

THE WHOLE FORMULA

The common mans' formula for sex consists of the five senses. This is only half of the formula. Until a couple have the whole formula, neither will feel good about the experience. It is much like trying to bake a cake without the leavening. To be satisfying requires the whole formula, not just half of it.

The general concept upon which society is built today is the concept that there is nothing but the physical. All science is built entirely upon the five senses of the physical world. Most people believe anything in the name of science is unquestionable. Most of the famous scientists have believed there was something more. They have tried long and hard to measure it with their physical instruments. Some have come close enough to prove there is something more here, but what is it? Their instruments cannot tell them, because what they are looking for is not of this physical world.

To a small extent what is missing is obvious to all of us. We are all aware of the emotions; love, hate, fear, jealousy and anger. They come from the subconscious. They are not of this physical world. Love is not related to the five senses

It is a well known fact that the subconscious is huge, much larger than the conscious. It is like an iceberg, almost all hidden. The more we study it, the less we seem to know of it. The emotions are somewhere within it. Scientists still cannot explain why an instantaneous change of emotion will instantly and drastically change the body's electrical resistance, but it is well known that it does and the principle is commonly used, such as in the lie detector and similar devices.

The "placebo effect" is well known and medical science knows the placebo effect is as powerful as their strong medications. No drug test can be accepted until the placebo effect can be proven not to be a factor in the testing. It has been demonstrated to suddenly cure the most sever of sicknesses, even cancer. But what is it? It is a function of the subconscious. That seems to be agreed upon. If we could control it we might eliminate much sickness. Science cannot control it or explain it. Nor can they deny it.

This only demonstrates that there is a whole other world science cannot reach. Even the hypnotist can only reach a small part of the subconscious, although he may be able to demonstrate some very dramatic effects of it. The physical is the only part science can reach. Many spiritual leaders have always told us there is much more here than scientists can explain.

Some say the subconscious is the most powerful thing on earth. Any way you look at it, the subconscious is very influential and mysterious. Most of the functions of the body are controlled by it, such as breathing, our heartbeat and hundreds and probably thousands of other things. The primary process of learning to drive a car or ride a bicycle are largely processes of training the subconscious mind. After that, they become largely automatic.

It sometimes seems that the subconscious can overpower the basic laws of physics. It has been demonstrated by hypnotists that a lighted match can be placed under a finger of a person under deep hypnoses which would ordinarily produce a very severe burn and if the person is told it is ice, the person will have no burn at all after they come out of hypnoses! It is a matter of what the subconscious perceives it as! Do not experiment with this unless you are a professional hypnotist.

Think of your sexual pleasure. You have to be in a state of sexual excitement before the stimulations become pleasurable. There are many things going on in your subconscious before it can become pleasurable.

Likewise there are many things that influence a woman's subconscious attitudes toward sex and thus her physical experiences. If she has grown up hearing her mother discussing sex with her friends as though her father was only using her mother, and the other women discussing it similarly while they receive no pleasure from it, she will have a hard time enjoying it herself. Even if she has an orgasm, she will very likely not enjoy it. The orgasm may be very real, but she will not feel any pleasure from it. If her mother and father both enjoyed sex together she will probably easily find pleasure in it.

If her first experience of sex is unpleasant, her belief that men only use women for sex will be substantiated and hard to change.

Most women can enjoy sex much more than any man if she will relax and experience it with an open mind, provided you take the time to give it to her. If you really care for her as a person you can also experience much pleasure in giving it to her through your awareness of her responses. You can sense her physical feelings and her feelings toward you when giving her these extended pleasures. You should enjoy giving the pleasure to her as well as enjoying her body much more than in simple sex alone.

Having sex with Miss America is not necessarily that great of an experience. Personal attraction, personality and mutual rapport are the important things. It is her response to your love making which is important to you. Does she smile? Do her eyes brighten? Does she make genuine sounds of pleasure? Does she kiss passionately? Does she pull you to her? Does she run her hands over your body?

For all of these reasons it is VERY important that a woman's first sexual experience be very pleasant. Always speak to her and in front of her as making love WITH her, never to her. Never say or imply that you need sex and she should give it to you. Never say "I need you", referring to your sexual needs. If you take the time to give her the extensive pleasure she is capable of, you will quickly develop a better relationship than you can imagine, while she will gladly satisfy your sexual needs and share them with you.

If a baby is conceived in an act of love between the two parents, the love will be passed on to the baby and the love of the baby will most likely be expressed by both parents after the baby is born and growing up. If it is conceived as an accident and not wanted, it will subconsciously know that. If it is conceived intentionally by two partners who have only a convenient relationship, the child will not get the love it needs. Every baby deserves this love from the moment of conception. If it is conceived in an act of quick momentary desire and relief, the baby will be more difficult to actually love.

There is no doubt that the emotions are centered in the subconscious and that they play a very important part in all of our lives.

So, the formula for "Love-Making" ceases to be "Sex", which is only half of the formula and is: "SEX+LOVE"= man+woman = the five senses+emotions.

The final formula has a magical effect and power not explainable by science.

CHAPTER 5

SEDUCTION

Seduction is usually considered to mean the art of removing a woman's clothing and getting her into the sex act. It is often thought of and practiced as tricking a woman. However, proper seduction is actually a two way communication between a man and woman, with both wanting the same things.

So how do the two of you first decide to have sex? The way it has largely been thought of over the centuries is a couple gets married and on their wedding night they are expected to have sex. The new wife sometimes had no idea of what was coming and was shocked. The husband often had to explain to her what her "wifely duties" were. Sex was one of her duties as a wife, like cooking and cleaning. It was often thought to be a sin for a woman to want or enjoy sex. She belonged to him, including her body and was his servant.

She often chose her husband or he was chosen for her only on the consideration of keeping the two families wealth safe or for his potential for supporting her well and the respect he commanded in the community. She was largely led to believe these were the main differences among men.

Very likely sex was a rudimentary act that did not do anything to bring them closer. He may have maintained a mistress who did know something of sex and enjoyed it. Fortunately, in more recent times the situation has improved considerably for both partners. However, the remnants of those times are still with us. Husbands are still often chosen for their ability to support her.

A man may do a woman a lot of favors and then thinks she will like him and want to date him. Then he's shocked when her date pulls up and she takes off with her date while he's repairing her car. But favors are for friendship and love is a different thing.

If you are on a date with her and wondering why she is not ready to jump in bed with you like they do in the movies, you may resort to something like: "All couples do it. That's what couples are all about. Don't you like me?" She will quite likely give into this. But don't get the idea she likes this. I have had several women complain to me about their sex with a guy they are dating. When I ask them why they do it if it is unpleasant, the answer is always the same: "That's what he expects." What a poor excuse! What a poor relationship! How different is this from the old concept that sex was the wife's duty, the pleasure of which was not to be shared by her?

Working up to sex should be a two party activity, just as sex itself should be. Remember, it takes two to tango, but generally the man leads, the woman follows. She must follow closely or the dance will not go well. But leading is a skill in love making as it is in dancing, and she will not follow unless you are actually leading. But she must be following. If she is not there will be no dance.

She must be enjoying the dance or she will not dance. Although he is leading, to really go well she must be expressing herself continually. This is not male chauvinism. No matter how much women complain about it, it is actually a woman's nature. She wants the man to lead.

Occasionally, the woman may take the lead. She may kiss you by surprise. She may take the lead half the time and that is usually a great experience if she does. If she does and you are interested in her, do not hesitate to respond quickly with enthusiasm. If you are really interested in her and you are caught off guard and hesitate, she will get the impression you really don't care for her or you are just not a lover. You must respond to any leads she takes as well as her responses to your leads. If she takes the lead, you probably have already missed her signals to come ahead.

Even if she takes the lead at times, you can still adapt most of this book to make the experience what both of you really want. She may accept fifteen minute sex, but that is not likely what she actually wants.

This book is primarily based upon the more typical situation in which you will need to take the lead. In some situations, you may have to play the game by ear, so to speak, as it unfolds. However, the following will be very helpful.

Although women may take an active part in sex, their basic nature is to completely relax and enjoy the feelings, not caring where the feelings are coming from or what you are doing to her as long as it is pleasant. A man must purposefully and actively create those feelings in her.

Still, although you are leading, you must be following her readiness for the next step and her desire for it. If you are not following her in that way, you will very likely fall flat on your face. You must have a feeling of what she is enjoying and what she is not.

When is she getting bored with what she previously really liked? What kind of sounds is she making? Why? Is she smiling faintly? Are her eyes bright or very relaxed? Is she pulling you closer? Is she pushing you away? Is that expression on her face an expression of pleasure or displeasure?

She may naturally put her hand on your upper arm and squeeze your arm. If she does not, take her hand and put it there. Now she will probably squeeze your arm tighter when she is enjoying your love making most and her hand will probably begin to relax as she begins to get bored by what you are doing. This is the time to move to the next step. In this way she is leading you. She may not realize she is doing so. You can judge her feelings in other ways. Is her breathing tense? How about her facial expression?

When she relaxes in these ways she is ready to move on. By these things she is leading you.

If you simply establish a routine, it will bore both of you. Each episode should be spontaneous. You must both be leading and following and aware of the other one, but in different ways.

The purpose of this book is to make a good and safe experience for both of you. Always remember that when it gets to the point of actual sex, she should have almost lost control of herself. She is completely relaxed and just enjoying the pleasure you are giving her. She is not thinking. She has already placed herself almost completely in trust to you. She really does not want to think about exactly what you are doing to her. Only that it feels good and she is enjoying it. She honestly often does not know nor care what you are doing to her.

For this reason, it is imperative that you take the responsibility to protect her from pregnancy and diseases. Without realizing what has been happening she has gradually been moved from having no idea of what is coming, into full sex and she may still not realize exactly what is happening. She is not in a position at any stage to make an intelligent decision about such things as birth control. It is your responsibility unless you have discussed it before hand, which is doubtful the first time. If you say; "How about having sex tonight?" she will probably answer that with a slap, even though she was already expecting to have sex with you.

Always remember: If you get her pregnant, you will probably be in for 19 years of child support and maybe supporting her also, even if not married to her! Also remember that if she says; "It's O.K. I'm on the pill"; if she forgets to take it exactly at the right time, just once, she may get pregnant and you will be legally and financially responsible, even if she did consent to it. Yes, even if you have found too many differences between the two of you and never want to see her again.

Furthermore, there are many women who want a baby but do not really like men, do not want to get married and do not want a lover. They are looking for a father and maybe a lifetime of support. They are often the easiest to get in bed and the easiest to get into the sex act. They WANT to get pregnant! They usually do not enjoy sex. But they pretend to like it until they get pregnant. The ten minute sex with a lubricant is fine for her. Never forget that! Her consent to the sex will not change your responsibilities. Birth control is your responsibility. Always use a condom, no matter what time of month it is for her.

CHAPTER 6

MAKING LOVE TOGETHER

Making love with a woman properly is not a matter of tricking her. It is a matter of giving her what she wants, and often what she does not know she wants. It is somewhat of a game and you may find you enjoy the game as much as she does. Like any game, you have to learn the game. This is a game where you direct it.

She must participate and play the game however. Like any game, if she is not interested in playing the game, there will be no game. You can easily tell if she is interested. If you want to play a game with someone you must suggest playing the game. Seduction is no different, but you will not ask her verbally, you will ask her through physical invitation.

Women really hate to be asked if they can be kissed or otherwise approached. She may be ready for a kiss and wanting it, but if you ask her if you can, she will likely say no and quite possibly turn cool. To ask a woman if you may do something to her is a clear sign to her that you are not in rapport with her. You should be able to tell when a woman wants to be kissed or wants to be otherwise approached by her bright eyes, pleasant mood and body language in general. When you think the time is right and she is giving you the right body language you will have to try it. If you are wrong, she will let you know.

A "no" in any language is not a final answer. She may say "no" a half dozen times while she is building up to a strong "yes". Or she may enjoy your pursuit of her, but not be ready to go further. Or she may just be enjoying your pursuit because it builds her self confidence and is enjoyable building her ego while she has no interest in you. Now I will tell you how to lead her into love and sex.

When you meet someone you find really attractive, you need to let her know you find her especially attractive right away. As time goes by it is much more difficult to convince her. If she labels you as a friend, then that is what you will be. If she has labeled you as a potential lover, you have a good chance. You can still just be friends with no problem if you decide to. But if she has labeled you as a friend you will have a hard time ever being her lover.

First impressions are lasting impressions. You do not need to plan on seducing her at this point. Just talking to her and exchanging a few friendly flirtations is it's own reward. If you think you might want to be her lover, be sure she does not label you as a friend before you decide.

Once you get to know her you may definitely decide you do not want to know her any better or in an intimate way. That is no problem. But the two of you can still enjoy some friendly flirtation before you have decided you would like to have sex with her or after you have both decided it will not go any farther. If you have known her a while without expressing her attractiveness and suddenly realize you find her particularly desirable, you may have to work at it a lot more. The following is if you want to be labeled as her lover.

The game usually starts with a simple "Hi", "Hello" or what is appropriate to the situation.. If you are being introduced and she has returned the greeting you might respond with something such as; "My pleasure". Your accent should reinforce your words. In many cases just getting her into a friendly conversation, finding out her name and a few things about her is a form of flirtation and about all you can do. Sometimes after meeting her you might take her hand or upper arm and lead her to the punch bowl or such.

You must seem at ease and natural to her. It you stammer and hesitate in what you are talking about, she will feel you are already not at ease with her, that you are thinking hard on what to say and what not to say and you are artificial. This is usually worse than saying the wrong thing. Relax and be yourself.

Now if you are finding her body especially attractive, you need to let her know you do. There is one strange thing about women: Almost all of them, including the most attractive and the most conceited, are very concerned and insecure about their attractiveness, including their outward appearance. A woman who is perfect by all common standards will be very concerned about a very small mole or pimple, while another woman will place such a mark in the same place with make up!

It is usually better not to bluntly tell her how attractive she is at first. That seems fake. But let her know you find her physically very attractive by letting her see you looking over her body and show some signs of not being able to avoid looking at it. Do not stop and look over her whole body at once.

Look her in the eye first with some look of excitement and pleasure in your face while carrying on a conversation. Now look at her breasts if they are prominently displayed. Don't stare at them. Just a quick look at them while she is looking you in the eye as if you cannot resist the look. A second look a minute latter is in order, but do not stare. You are trying to avoid looking, right? But she has them on display does she not? How can you help but look?

Look her face over and her hair. As soon as you are positioned to do so, look her whole body over and be sure she sees you doing so, but do not stare. Spend most of your time looking into her eyes for short periods of time, then away while talking, but not starring her in the eye and show some excitement or pleasure in your face. Now tell her she is very attractive or better, how certain of her qualities are very attractive to you if you can bring it into the conversation somewhat naturally. Some flirtatious remarks are in order, but usually nothing directly sexy.

Look to see what kind of jewelry she is wearing or some message on a T-shirt. This may give you further excuses to look at her breasts with her knowing it. These are things she is displaying for attraction and conversation. Be sure you take advantage of them. Is she really interested in the subject on her T-shirt? Was she really there? Does she wish she had been? Does the jewelry have a story behind it? Is that her astrological sign? If so when is her birthday?

Find out as much about her from your conversations as possible without getting overly personal. If she mentions some sport or activity she likes or is interested in, if you are too, say so, but do not try to sell yourself by pretending to like what you don't. That will catch up with you later. Mostly listen to her attentively and respond intelligently. Carry half the conversation but not much more. Listen to her. At this point you must express your attraction to her personality; to her as a person.

The next time you meet her try to pick up on the last conversation, something that will show her you really were listening and she is important. Every time you pass her close enough at least say a quick "Hi" and show by your face it is a pleasure. Just touch her arm if you get close enough but be careful in surprising her from behind. This is frightening to many women. If you get her attention from a distance, give her some sign you see her, such as a big smile while looking her in the eye. Maybe even a wink.

From the beginning, flirtation is in order. Flirtation often takes many forms. Sometimes it is just getting her attention. It often takes the form of suggestions that can be in the form of a joke, or something that can be interpreted as sexy, but also in another interesting way. One way may be very sexy, but the other way must be otherwise and bring both to mind by suggestion, a pun. The sexy interpretation should be something you would not say directly and must be something she can pass off as a joke, even though she gets the message and enjoys it. It is often something she would be very embarrassed or even highly offended to openly acknowledge its possible meaning as sexually oriented. A flirtation may also be a comment expressing an appreciation of some part of her body, but should not be too directly sexual. If she returns your flirtations, you can then make them stronger and more direct.

Flirtation is also your body language. That is a whole extensive subject in it self. Pay close attention to hers.

Begin touching her very politely as soon as possible, on your first meeting. In a few situations a hug is appropriate as a first greeting. In some situations you could ask her to dance with your hand on her back or waist and holding her hand. Or you might guide her through a door you have opened for her with your hand on her back or waist. You might take her hand or upper arm and take her to the punch bowl or other place. You might even ask her to dance a slow dance with you which will give you a full body contact with your cheek to hers! In a group, touching her arm to get her attention is in order. At least touch her shoulder or arm or the back of the hand quickly when parting from her as a farewell gesture. If you appear uncomfortable in touching her, she will know you are not at ease with her and this will be a big turnoff.

Some people are touching people and communicate very largely through touching. Others are much more reluctant to touch. If she talks fast, she probably communicates more by visual contact. She will talk about how she saw or sees things or how things look. She will not be quite as easy to touch, but must be touched. If she talks slower and uses largely words of sound such as "That sounds good"; "It was music to my ears" etc. she probably responds strongly to music, voices and other sounds and such verbal expressions in conversation. She will be easier to touch than if she is visual. If she talks still slower and tends to look down, she almost certainly is a feeling person and will want polite touching immediately and polite touching continuously. She will talk about how things feel. She will want slow soft conversation with feeling and polite touching.

If you get a date with her, an intimate kiss at some moment during the evening at some special time when she has responded more than usual to something you have said or something that has happened to excite both of you, will be easier and better received than the expected parting kiss at the door.

A date does not automatically include a kiss. But if things went well, at the end of a pleasant date it will probably include at least a somewhat intimate hug. This can be almost as good as a good kiss.

While hugging her, move on past her ear and kiss or gently nibble her neck toward the back. If she draws away, you are probably not making very intimate progress. If she pulls away but comes back with a smile, she is probably ready for a good kiss.

When you kiss her it is usually good to put your hand on her face as though to very gently hold her face in place while you kiss her. She will almost certainly like it. Don't you want to touch her smooth face gently? This will show her you are at ease with her and know women.

Once you have decided to seduce her, choose three "anchor" spots somewhere on her which you can easily touch anytime without it seeming strange or unusual, but which you will not touch accidently or at any time except when you want to arouse her sexually. Perhaps in the upper arm in a place and way you will not otherwise touch her, or maybe on the shoulder, or the back of her hand etc.

These must be touched in exactly the same way and pressure each time. Do not touch her here until she is in an orgasm, but plan it ahead of time.

Now choose three "anchor" words or sounds you will only use when you want to arouse her sexually in the future. These words should not seem out of place in normal conversation but cannot be a word you will use for any other purpose in conversation. Such words as "Wow!", "Ooh!" or such are good. These must always be spoken with exactly the same expression and loudness each time. It will not matter if other people use the same words in the same way with her. These words and touches will be tied to her by you. They can be spoken when in public without attracting any attention, but will bring to her mind what she was experiencing when you first anchored her (her orgasm). After an anchor word has been spoken she will be very much aroused.

An anchor is a subconscious association of something with something else. In this case it will be the height of her pleasure (an orgasm) with a touch or word you have chosen. In the future to bring that experience back to her, you will only have to touch her the way you have established at her anchor spot or use your anchor word and she will experience the same thing she was experiencing when you first anchored her. It will be very powerful, as when you remember your orgasm.

We use anchors quite often in our normal life. For instance our name is an anchor associating our name with us.

You should only use one anchor at a time, either an anchor word or an anchor spot. The word can even be used over the phone or in public or among friends. The touching anchor needs to be such that you can touch her in that place and manner while you are in a position to do so, while you are giving her that orgasm, as well as in everyday situations, such as among friends, so think ahead to what will be possible and best.

What you are going to do to seduce her is what she wants AT EACH MOMENT. Just as she wanted a kiss after some love making, but would not accept it before, she will want each step but only when she is ready, leading you through to the end of sex. She will not be ready for any of these advances until she was prepared by the previous step.

Once you have kissed her and she has responded with pleasure, hug her, nibble her neck, nibble her ear lobes but be very careful not to pull on her ear rings as they will be tender and it is easy to injure her ears. Keep returning to the kiss. Nibble on her lips. Keep the kiss moving slowly. Enter her mouth with your tongue only if she invites you by touching your tongue with hers first, while just barely moving your tongue through your lips. If she invites you in by touching your tongue with hers, then you can play with her tongue.

When each of these acts begins to get too repetitive, she may be desiring something more. You should be able to sense a reduction of her excitement from the last advance you made by her letting up with her grip of your arm, by a relaxing of her face, by a slowing and relaxing of her breathing, or a relaxing of her body in general, then its time to move on.

Start running your fingers and hands over her back and arms very lightly, and slowly, just barely touching the hair on her arms and body if there is any, or skin or through her clothing. If you are touching her through her clothing, use a very light touch, but enough that she can feel it. Move over all the areas you can politely reach. Keep kissing and hugging and show your pleasure. You are enjoying this, are you not?

Assuming she is showing signs of pleasure and excitement with this, when it is again seeming repetitious, you can try touching her breasts, perhaps as though accidentally at first. If she does not pull away from this you can feel the bottom of her breasts, perhaps only while hugging her with your arms on the bottom of her breasts possibly from behind at first. Then if she accepts this you may cup one hand and hold a breast in it, always very lovingly and as though you were holding the most precious thing in the world. Continue running your hands very lightly over her clothing and moving your hands around, coming back to the same places.

When this is all seeming repetitious to her, you may be able to move your hand up under her T-shirt or blouse or if you cannot do this, you may be able to unfasten her clothing so as to run your hand over her skin or breasts, perhaps through her bra. You can probably remove more of her clothing as each thing you do becomes too repetitious and accepted by her, as long as she seems to be enjoying it. How long each of these things take is difficult to tell. You may be able and want to move through these steps quickly or you may need to take quite a bit of time with some of them. Naturally, if all she is wearing is a bikini and top, she will probably be ready to move faster. It is up to her.

The whole idea is to only advance when she seems to be desiring more, not just when you want to. If what you are doing to her seems pleasant and increasingly pleasant to her, she will probably soon want more.

In this manner, you can probably remove all of her clothing, as she continues to expect you to remove her clothing in order to move her pleasure to new parts of her body, assuming you are in a place where she feels very safe from being intruded upon and not pressed for time. Remember to remove your own clothing as you remove hers. You are doing this together. To remove all of her cloths and keep yours on is a suggestion that you are dong something to her instead of with her.

CHAPTER 7

GETTING SERIOUS

In Chapter 6 you and she both ended up with all of your cloths off. If she came this far because each step was her desire, as it should have been, she is almost ready for sex. That does not mean intercourse. She is not ready for you to enter her. You need to develop a broader meaning of sex than is usually thought of. Remember: almost all of her body is her sex organ.

By now she should have a hand on one of your upper arms and is naturally squeezing it to express what she really feels, squeezing harder when she feels a deep pleasure and letting up a little as she becomes ready for more. This is natural to her. If she does not, take her hand and place it on your upper arm. She will probably just naturally squeeze your arm when she is feeling intense pleasure and let up as the pleasure lessons. When her grip on your arm lessons it is time to go further. This is a way of expressing herself that even the shyest woman will not feel embarrassed to express. If she does not squeeze it this way, you may be able to tell her to.

Now start with her neck and very lightly run your hands over her down to her knees. Kiss her whole body if you like. Continue running your hands over her whole body, or kissing it, but staying away from her pubic area at first. Start above her naval and moving downward and outward slowly.

It is good if she wants you to move faster and you hold back. Run your hands very lightly and slowly over her back and down to her knees but not into the crease between her buttocks. Stay away from her inner thighs. Now brush very lightly over her pubic hair just barely touching it. Go back to brushing over her entire body.

Be sure to come back and kiss her on the mouth and nibble her neck several times, while running your hand over her body. She will probably not give you a passionate kiss in return. Her awareness is on the pleasures of her body you are giving her. But kissing her gives her a feeling that you are giving her the pleasure because of her and not just because you want to touch her beautiful body, as almost any man would like to do.

Come back to the pubic hair a couple of more times. Always do everything as if it is what you want to do or cannot resist doing. Is it not? Her pleasure comes from the touching of her body, but also from the feeling that you are enjoying her body.

Come down to her clitoris and pass your hand over the hair very lightly. Go back and pass your hand over her body and legs again. Now, massage the heavy flesh almost covering the clitoris. She may or may not be aware she even has a clitoris. The clitoris is one of the most sensitive and pleasurable parts of her body. But don't start massaging it suddenly.

Now is the time to unroll a condom over your penis. If you have gone this far, you will almost certainly be able to go all the way. From now on you need to keep going without stopping or hesitating. You will not have time to stop and put your condom on.

Massage the flesh around the clitoris and gradually move inward toward her clitoris until you are very gently massaging the foreskin directly. Work slowly and keep her wanting more. Continue to massage the clitoris very gently but now move two fingers, down along the sides of it, inside of the labia minora, (the small lips protecting the clitoris) with more pressure than you are using to massage the foreskin of the clitoris.

The clitoris has a double shaft which you can feel passing under the two sides of this area. Massaging the two shafts and the head of the clitoris builds her excitement gradually higher and higher. Do not stop massaging the clitoris, but keep your fingers moving very lightly over it while massaging slightly harder and downward along the sides. Don't rush her as though you are impatient. Just keep giving her this pleasure. Speeding up will not increase her pleasure or take less time.

Her clitoris and her nipples are connected by the nerves very directly. They are closely connected but separate and different. Nibble or massage one of her nipples gently at the same time as the clitoris. She is really enjoying this and does not want to be rushed. Continue this without rushing it and after a while she will have an orgasm. Don't rush her orgasm. Just let her pleasure build higher and higher by itself. Once her orgasm begins (and you will know when it does) do not speed up.

Now whisper your first anchor word or sound. Do this for the first three times she has an orgasm in the clitoris. Speak your anchor word exactly the same way and volume as you will use in the future to arouse her. Do not use your touch anchor and word anchor during the same orgasm.

It is usually better not to tell her of these anchors, but it will not be a problem if she does know. Is this unfair or taking advantage of her? Actually, it is only reminding her of something she has enjoyed. It makes no demands on her. It is only increasing her pleasure and keeping her wanting more. If she has broken up with you and is no longer dating you it would be a violation of her former trust in you to again use any of these anchors in her presence.

If she is a virgin and has never been entered before, while she is in the middle of the first orgasm in her clitoris, enter her quickly. About one virgin in four will experience some pain the first time, occasionally but rarely she may experience considerable pain for a very short time. If she experiences pain while in the middle of an orgasm, she will experience the pain as extreme pleasure. If you do not know if she is a virgin or not, assume she is and follow this procedure.

Most boys wonder if they can find the hole to the vagina. It is not a problem. She has a raised lip around the clitoris and along the sides and back around the opening to the vagina, called the labia majora (See the figure in Chapter 2. If you place your penis between these lips and move forward, your penis will be guided to slide right into the vagina. You will probably have to press on it to enter. If she is a virgin, you could have to press hard. Do not hesitate. If she is a virgin, enter her quickly and then wait a couple of seconds to begin stroking slowly. Do not put your weight on her, you should support yourself.

If she is not a virgin and has been entered before, keep massaging her clitoris until she is through with that orgasm.

When that orgasm is finished her vagina is ready. It will help if she raises her legs to tilt her pelvis to a better angle for your penis. If she does not raise them, raise them for her.

When a woman is ready to be entered, she will almost always be very wet and the whole area including the inside of the vagina will be very wet and well lubricated. Her vagina will be heavily swollen with blood inside into a somewhat ribbed surface. This surface is very soft and moves when pressed on lightly. It is the gentile flow of blood through these swollen areas that feels so good to her when massaged.

If you enter her now, you will have completed your ejaculation and lost your erection before she more than starts her orgasm. You need to have your orgasm at the same time, together.

To accomplish this, Insert two fingers into her vagina and gently, slowly massage these soft swollen areas until she reaches a second orgasm, this time in the vagina. Be careful not to irritate her with your knuckles or fingernails or by putting a side pressure on her vaginal opening. Be sure your fingernails are short and sanded smooth so as not to injure her with them. Keep some pressure on the walls of the vagina with the fingers away from your nails.

This is a very different orgasm than the one in her clitoris and it feels very different to her.

Stroke steady without rushing. You will soon reach an orgasm yourself and hers will continue until yours has finished. While she is in this orgasm, use a different word or sound as an anchor for this orgasm.

When she reaches a vaginal orgasm, her vagina will come alive. Bringing her to an orgasm before you enter her will greatly increase your pleasure due to this activity in her vagina. Her orgasm will last until you are through. If you enter her without first bringing her to an orgasm by massaging the vagina with your fingers, she may not reach an orgasm until you are through and even then you will probably have to massage her vagina by hand to give her any orgasm. Both your greatest pleasure and hers will be in experiencing your extended orgasm at the same time as she is experiencing hers.

Many men think of their orgasm and their ejaculation as one and the same thing. If you do, your orgasm will probably be short and quick. You are trying to reach an orgasm because that is where the great pleasure is. When you do you then ejaculate as you believe this is part of the orgasm you are trying to achieve. When you ejaculate you will lose your erection. Your orgasm will be very short because your subconscious mind thinks it is supposed to produce your ejaculation at the same time as your orgasm begins.

Both you and your subconscious mind need to think of your orgasm and your ejaculation as two separate things, as they are. As you slowly make love to her your need to ejaculate slows down, while her readiness to have an orgasm speeds up.

The swollen ribbed vagina massages your penis perfectly and is warm with blood. Your penis massages this swollen interior, pushing the blood in and out of different areas. This is what feels so good to her. The active orgasm in her vagina also massages your penis, raising your level of pleasure still higher.

Once she has finished her orgasm in her vagina, this swelling can disappear almost instantly, leaving a large cavity in her vagina with a smooth, relatively hard surface. This is known as tenting. Once this has happened, she will no longer experience any pleasure in the vagina and you will probably not either. This will not likely happen before you ejaculate.

During intercourse, relax and enjoy the pleasure. Do not rush it. Never think your ejaculation will never come. It will, but it will no longer seem important. It is the orgasm that is important.

Soon after she reaches an orgasm in the vagina, her cervix will probably drop down hard over the vaginal opening and if you come out too close to the opening at this time while stroking, it may push you out. You may or may not be able to get back in. Therefore, be careful not to come out too close to the opening while stroking until you are finished.

CHAPTER 8

EXTENDED LOVE

Finished? She will probably think you are finished now and you both will feel satisfied. You can stop here if you want. However, after you have had sex with her the first time, you can give her a third orgasm in her "G spot". It is usually best not to try this the first time.

This should always be done only after her orgasm in the clitoris and can be done before or after intercourse. The clitoris must always be first. It prepares the rest. It can even be done after she has tented. See the Figure, Chapter 2, "Anatomy". The G spot is at the top front of her vagina about one inch inside the vagina. Your finger can just reach it while bent upward without putting pressure on her with a knuckle. She may or may not know she has such an area.

As you can see from the Anatomy Figure, this is above the urethra, deep in the flesh. Therefore this requires considerably more pressure than massaging the clitoris or vagina. Not enough pressure to be uncomfortable to her, of course, but it is not on the surface as the other areas of her pleasure are and she probably wants quite a bit of pressure there. Start massaging the area and move around a little until she suddenly reacts. Then you have found it.

Once you have located it, slowly massage it until she has an orgasm and finishes the orgasm. This may be her strongest orgasm. She will probably not be as relaxed with this experience as with the clitoris or vagina. She will probably be more aware and she may tell you how hard she wants it and where.

Now use a different word or sound to anchor her a third time in this third area. Use all three of these anchor words or sounds at least three times in three different experiences.

Then, when having sex after those three times, use the three places you have chosen to touch her with her cloths on and can easily touch her the same way and pressure while she is in her orgasm. Touch her three times in these places during three more experiences of future sex. These should be places that will not seem strange to touch her.

In the future, you can bring a full memory of any orgasm in which you have anchored her, to back to her, by speaking one of the words or touching one of her anchors, even over the phone or in public or among friends, without anyone noticing and without her even knowing why this memory is coming to her at this time.

In this way you can keep the three kinds of orgasms coming to her mind whenever you wish.

If you really want to please her, once she is finished with her orgasm in the vagina, and the G-spot you can give her "Extended Love". To do so, go back to the clitoris and start all over. Although she will not yet be ready for any more in the vagina or the G-spot, by now she will be fully ready to experience more pleasure in the clitoris. After another orgasm in the clitoris, she will be ready to experience another orgasm in the vagina or G spot.

It does not take her long to prepare to do it again, like a man does. She will be able to repeat this full cycle until she is exhausted if she likes and if her lover will give it to her. It will be just as strong each time. As it passes through each area of her body, it will change drastically, so it is not boring to her. It is a continuous flow of sensations. Love making between these cycles of her orgasms will also be well received and let her know you are not through. It is doubtful that you will be able to get an erection again, although you may. If not you will have to massage the vagina entirely by hand.

In the average woman this will be about fifty total minutes of orgasm! There will also be some time between. Some will want still more and some less. The better physical condition she is in, the more pleasure she will be able to experience.

And so it is that she has three places she can experience an orgasm in, each separate and each feeling different from the others. As she goes through the cycle, the experience is continually changing for her. It is not one long boring pleasure for her. Now you have learned to play this fine instrument. With practice you can learn to play more complex melodies.

Now do you see why she can have more pleasure in sex than any man?

After you have had sex with her the first time, starting from the beginning, she will probably want to go through all that you did the first time, but much faster. After you have anchored her as described above, every time you touch your anchor spot on her or you use your anchor word in exactly the same way you originally did, her subconscious will bring her back to experiencing what she was feeling when you anchored her! By using these anchors several times in the hour or two before you start actually making love to her, you will greatly accelerate her preparedness for sex.

The anchor word can be spoken over the phone or any other place to highly arouse her. The touch or the word can be used while you are among friends, or in public without anyone knowing it. Using your anchor word on her is building her up to sex without even touching her. In this way you can keep her ready for sex and the sex she will be thinking of will be with you. She is fully tied to you personally by the anchors you have created, not to anybody else.

Just because you have had sex with her and have anchored her is no reason not to touch her commonly in other ways or to stop flirting with her. It is all important to preparing her for sex and to maintain and build your relationship.

After you have had sex with her the first time, try to get her to talk to you freely of her experience and get her to talk to you before the next experience of sex about what she likes and what she does not if she will. She may be too shy to do so. Don't push her. Never speak to her of sex as a dirty subject, something sinful or something funny. Always speak of it as a wonderful experience the two of you went through together. You can share sexy jokes and stories and laugh at them. The sex should be playful, but the sex between you is not funny.

Make it clear to her that you want to be told when you are doing something she does not like and what you can do that she will like better. You want to please her. Every woman is different and what I have explained here is what women commonly like and will accept. This is usually the best for your first time.

The first time is hardly the time to plan ahead together.

Every one is different and as you learn what your woman likes, the sex can greatly improve for both of you. You can tell her what she can do to make it better for you and what you would like but be careful about getting kinky unless she gives some indications she might like it. Never tell her what you expect from her. You can tell her what turns you on and what you enjoy. But do not tell her she owes it to you to do this or that. What you like may offend her and she does not owe it to you to do anything that she finds offensive.

If she is ready to talk about it and plan ahead, it is good to plan for her to remain fully aware during one episode so she can let you know what she likes that you are doing, what she does not like and what she would like instead, if she knows what she would like. She may not know. You may not know some things you like. Some experimentation may be needed.

After this, you can tell her you would like for her to tell you of any changes she would like to try at any time in the future, either always or occasionally.

For things she does not like, she can usually just push your hand away, push you away or hold your hand so as to lighten or increase your pressure to show she wants it differently or how she likes it. For things she would like, she may be able to put your hand where she would like it, tighten her hold on your arm or pull you to her.

Sex should always be fun, relaxed and playful for both of you, just as playing any game, sport, dancing or other activity or just walking hand in hand. It should never be a solemn experience, but one of mutual pleasure and fun.

Once actual sex has begun, conversation is usually distracting. On the other hand telling her what you love about her and her body is great, especially when running your hands over her body and viewing it, or kissing her without expecting a kiss in return. Low, slow soft words are the words of love. You can continue with this throughout, as long as she knows she does not have to answer or even listen if she does not want to. If she is not listening or replying to your conversation, it is no insult. She is just deep into her feelings, which is where you want her.

Remember that she will go into a completely relaxed state of just experiencing the pleasure. When she reaches an orgasm she will go into a slight or wild muscle spasm. She does not want to be disturbed from any of this by conversation or anything else. But even if she is not listening, her subconscious mind most certainly is.

So you see, she will seldom enjoy simple intercourse, with no orgasm or with her one orgasm suddenly cut short. She will probably have to be coerced into it the next time. How long will that last? Will she and her lover have a really good relationship if he continually yanks her special meal (her orgasm) out from under her face after each first bite?

Hopefully she will show some signs of positive response and passion as soon as you kiss her or before. This will be by taking an active part in your kiss, showing some noticeable positive reaction to having her neck nibbled, running her hands over your body as you are running your hands over hers, running her fingers through your hair and/or drawing you closer when hugging or squeezing your hand. These are usually her ways of telling you what she wants. Pay attention. She probably wants what she is giving. That is what she assumes you want too. If she does not show any signs of affection toward you after you have had sex with her, you may never have a satisfactory relationship.

It is your responsibility to give her the pleasure she is capable of experiencing. It is her responsibility to show you her feelings of pleasure and affection and appreciation for you and your efforts and give you some of the special pleasures you are capable of, although nothing that offends her. You and your body needs loving too. Not just sex. She should do this because she wants to, not because it is her duty.

If she has not been holding your arm in such a way as to let you know what she is feeling by squeezing your arm tighter when she is really feeling a strong pleasure and letting up on your arm when she is ready for something more, you should suggest to her that she do so.

CHAPTER 9

GREAT SEX IN 50 MINUTES

Most people in this rushing age will not want to spend the time for Extended Love and most men especially will want to get through sex quickly as they have throughout history.

However, using some of the knowledge in this book, he can increase his pleasure, often considerably, with very little extra time and effort, while completely satisfying his mate. That is the goal of this chapter.

When first seducing a new lover, most men will take quite a bit of time, perhaps even taking a week end vacation or longer with her. If he will follow the basics of this book up through that extra time, even though it is only three hours, he can have her anchored in the clitoris. Thereafter, he can bring her to a climax in the clitoris in 35 minutes after using his anchors, even over the telephone or while out with friends.

The clitoris is the only proper approach to the vagina. Stimulating it is what lubricates her, and causes it to swell inside. She may lubricate sufficiently without it, but sometimes she will not.

By using your anchors on her an hour or two before sex, even over the phone and during the beginning of love making, you can quickly prepare her for sex. A couple of passionate kisses, nibble her neck and hold her tight, use your anchors on her again and she will be ready for you to stimulate her clitoris and she can complete that orgasm in a few minutes.

Now, after her orgasm in her clitoris, if you insert two fingers into her vagina and massage it for a few minutes, she will reach an orgasm there and if you enter her now, her vagina will feel alive and your pleasure will be greatly increased over what it would be if you only kissed her a couple of times, hugged her, added a lubricant and entered her.

If you ejaculate in six minutes or less you need to do something about it. You are cutting both yourself and her short. See Chapter 7 for ways to correct this. If you prefer, a Neuro-Linguistic Programmer can usually cure your problem quickly and usually will not be very expensive. Go to the web and find one in your area.

You need to separate your concept of your orgasm from your concept of your ejaculation. They are two different things. If you think of them as one and the same thing your ejaculation will probably happen as soon as you begin your orgasm and its' all over for both of you. You can experience a lot more pleasure than that.

Now you have experienced your maximum of physical pleasure and she is satisfied too. You have considerably improved the pleasure for both of you.

CHAPTER 10

OTHER ISSUES

Both men and woman build a sexual tension through there body as there desire builds up to sex. This tension is relieved by an orgasm. If a woman repeatedly builds up this tension and this tension is not relieved by an orgasm, she will often become nervous and tense without knowing why. She may also become hungry for the orgasm to release it. Her subconscious mind will often interpret this hunger for an orgasm as a hunger for food. But as she eats to satisfy the hunger, the hunger will not be satisfied and she may continue to eat compulsively and not be able to control her eating. She may start putting on excessive weight as a result. All overweight is not caused by this, of course, but a lot is.

Look how many young girls are nice and thin and how many of them start putting on excessive weight as they mature. You don't see nearly as much overweight developing among men in the 20 year old range. And yet there is little doubt that women try harder to keep their weight down than the men. Is it because she needs an orgasm to satisfy her hunger? Maybe.

Furthermore, this unreleased tension affects the body in many other ways. There is good reason to believe that this nervous tension can cause headaches and contribute to many illnesses that seem entirely unrelated. Several books have been written concerning the effects of the subconscious mind on illness and disease. Dissatisfaction of the subconscious mind for various reasons can be extremely dangerous. We are supposed to be happy.

In relation to putting on weight, scientific studies have shown that sex requires more energy than any other common activity and for this reason alone sexually active women tend to have less overweight problems than others. This is especially true of those practicing Extended Love.

The average woman can experience about fifty minutes of actual ever changing orgasm in one session of sex. Some as much as seventy-five minutes. A man seldom more than ten. An orgasm consumes huge amounts of energy in both men and women. A man is exercising hard in a different way, and he is undergoing considerable exertion other than his orgasm. A woman is usually very passive. But her orgasm is not.

An orgasm produces heavy exercise in many muscles. In a woman, the three orgasms are different and some different muscles are involved. If she is having fifty minutes of orgasms twice a week in the three parts of her body, it will go a long way toward keeping her thin, trim and alive.

There is no doubt but what Extended Love helps keep people to stay in good physical health.

So, when he went down to meet his buddies after rolling off of her, did he really; "Fuck her good?" If so, he will not have to brag about it to strengthen his ego. He will know if he did.

CHAPTER 11

IS SHE ABNORMAL?

A survey was taken of couples that had been in a steady sexual relationship for more than six months. The results were quite interesting.

39% of the men said they used a lubricant. Only one out of eight women reported that they achieved more than the beginning of an orgasm before her lover was finished. The average time for foreplay before intercourse was 20 minutes.

More than half of the men believed their lovers were abnormal in not being able to reach an orgasm with them.

Only one fifth of the women believed they were abnormal in not reaching an orgasm with their mate.

So in twenty minutes of foreplay she was not sufficiently lubricated. Until she is properly naturally lubricated, her vagina is almost certainly not swollen properly and he will be entering her in a condition where her vagina is not prepared to massage his penis satisfactorily, so he cannot be experiencing the pleasure he should be.

The man and woman are not synchronized. He is loosing his erection by the time she is getting started and she needs at least another ten minutes. These are the reasons she must have her orgasm in the clitoris before the vagina is ready.

However, she is still not ready to reach an orgasm with him or at all without some additional help.

That is why I recommend massaging the vagina before entering her. Then his orgasm will come with hers and both partners will experience their orgasm together and both will have a better experience if he does. Her orgasm will still be going when he is through. Some men who love their mate massage her vagina after they are through to finish the orgasm she has just started and wants. This is O.K., but the two are not reaching an orgasm together this way, which would be better for both.

I have had several men say something to me to the effect of: "Are you trying to tell me my penis is not what she needs?"

This is certainly a good question. The answer is, it is what she needs, she just needs more of it. But how is the man to give her more of it?

Some resort to anesthetizing the penis. This prevents his ejaculation and gives her what she needs. However, you cannot anesthetize it for ten minutes and then suddenly start feeling what you should be. So now the man is not receiving his pleasure and will not be satisfied.

A few will strap on a plastic penis over their own and use it to bring her to an orgasm and then remove the plastic penis to complete their orgasm together. This is O.K. if you like.

How can we explain why the man and woman are out of sync with each other? That is a problem.

Women usually need about an hour and a half of foreplay to be ready. This can be considerably reduced with the use of the anchors. Then she has a clitoris. It needs to be massaged to give her an orgasm before she is really ready to be entered.

The clitoris cannot be massaged with the penis. What then is it for? We may have a hard time explaining that. Whether we understand why, it makes no difference. It is an important part of her and her sexual experience. It needs to be manually massaged. We cannot deny or ignore that. We may not be able to understand that. It seems that only the one who designed her can fully understand all of these things.

We can only know the realities and work with them.

But if her lover will accept her as she is and himself as he is, he can work with them to the satisfaction of both.

If he will start using his anchors on her two hours before beginning love play and continue to do so at least two more times until he begins to massage her clitoris, he can reduce the foreplay she wants from the hour and a half, down to thirty minutes and give her two good orgasms in a total of fifty minutes while also improving his experience.